LIVER DETOX
SMOOTHIE RECIPES

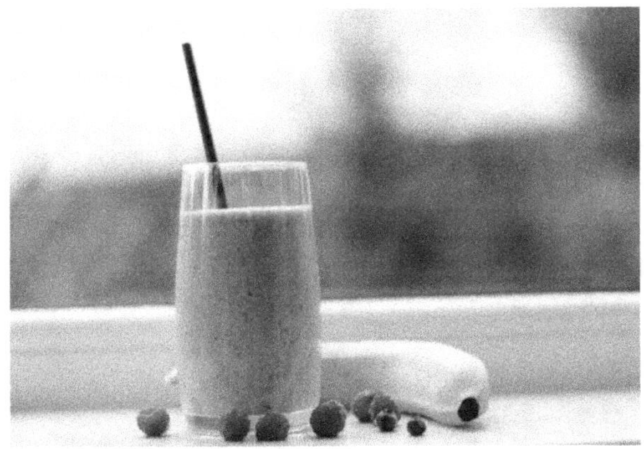

DR. JESSICA SMITH

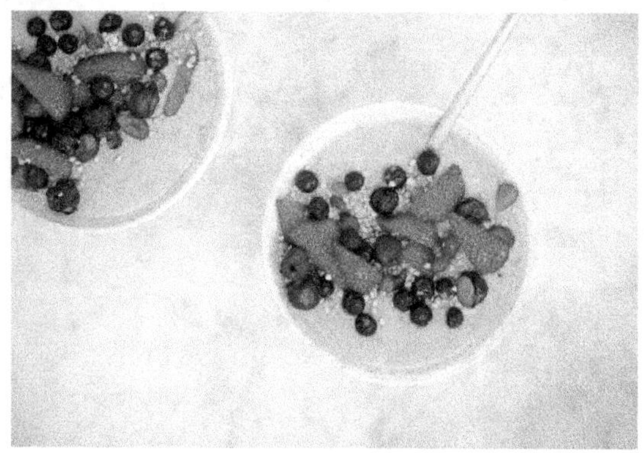

TABLE OF CONTENTS

CHAPTER ONE

How to Use this Cookbook

Gather Ingredients: Collect all the necessary ingredients for your liver detox smoothie. This typically includes fruits, vegetables, leafy greens, and additional detoxifying ingredients like ginger, turmeric, or lemon.

Wash Produce: Thoroughly wash all fruits, vegetables, and greens to remove any dirt, pesticides, or contaminants.

Prepare Ingredients: Peel and chop fruits and vegetables as needed to fit into your blender.

Choose Your Recipe: Select a liver detox smoothie recipe that appeals to you and aligns with your dietary preferences and goals. There are many variations available, so choose one that includes ingredients you enjoy.

Blend Ingredients: Add all the prepared ingredients to your blender. Start with the liquid base, such as water, coconut water, or almond milk, followed by the fruits, vegetables, and any additional ingredients.

Adjust Consistency: Blend the ingredients until smooth. If the smoothie is too thick, you can add more liquid to achieve your desired consistency.

Taste Test: Once blended, taste the smoothie to ensure it meets your flavor preferences. You can adjust the sweetness or tartness by adding more fruits or a splash of citrus juice if needed.

Serve Immediately: Pour the liver detox smoothie into glasses and serve immediately to enjoy its freshness and nutritional benefits fully.

Optional Additions: If desired, you can enhance your liver detox smoothie with additional toppings or garnishes such as chia seeds, hemp seeds, or a sprinkle of cinnamon.

Enjoy Regularly: Incorporate liver detox smoothies into your regular routine for optimal results. Enjoy them as a refreshing and nourishing beverage to support liver health and overall well-being.

Remember to consult with a healthcare professional before making significant changes to your diet, especially if you have any existing health conditions or concerns.

Understanding liver detox smoothies involves grasping their role in supporting liver health and overall well-being.

The liver plays a crucial role in detoxifying the body by filtering out toxins, metabolizing nutrients, and producing bile to aid in digestion.

However, factors like poor diet, environmental toxins, and excessive alcohol consumption can burden the liver, leading to sluggishness and compromised function.

Liver detox smoothies are specifically crafted to provide a concentrated dose of nutrients that support liver function and promote detoxification.

These smoothies typically contain ingredients rich in antioxidants, vitamins, and minerals, such as leafy greens, fruits, and herbs known for their detoxifying properties.

For example, leafy greens like kale and spinach are packed with chlorophyll, which can aid in toxin removal, while fruits like berries and citrus provide a potent dose of vitamin C, supporting liver detoxification pathways.

Additionally, liver detox smoothies may include ingredients like ginger, turmeric, and beets, known for their anti-inflammatory and liver-supporting properties.

These ingredients work synergistically to help the liver eliminate toxins more efficiently and reduce inflammation, promoting overall liver health.

Incorporating liver detox smoothies into your diet can be a convenient and delicious way to support your liver's natural detoxification processes and enhance your overall health and vitality.

However, it's essential to remember that while liver detox smoothies can be beneficial, they should complement a balanced diet and healthy lifestyle choices for optimal results.

Always consult with a healthcare professional before starting any new dietary regimen, especially if you have underlying health conditions or concerns.

Principles of Liver Detox Smoothie

The principles of liver detox smoothies revolve around utilizing nutrient-dense ingredients that support liver function and promote detoxification. These principles guide the creation of smoothie recipes aimed at optimizing liver health and overall well-being.

Firstly, liver detox smoothies prioritize ingredients rich in antioxidants, vitamins, and minerals.

These nutrients help neutralize harmful free radicals and support the liver's detoxification pathways. Ingredients such as leafy greens (e.g., kale, spinach), fruits (e.g., berries, citrus), and herbs (e.g., cilantro, parsley) are commonly included for their antioxidant properties.

Secondly, liver detox smoothies focus on incorporating ingredients with anti-inflammatory properties.

Chronic inflammation can impair liver function, so ingredients like ginger, turmeric, and omega-3 fatty acids from sources like flaxseed or chia seeds are often included to help reduce inflammation and promote liver health.

Thirdly, liver detox smoothies emphasize hydration and fiber intake. Adequate hydration supports liver function by aiding in the elimination of toxins, while fiber helps promote regular bowel movements and the removal of waste products from the body.

Finally, liver detox smoothies aim for balance and variety. By incorporating a diverse range of ingredients, smoothies can provide a wide array of nutrients that support overall health and well-being.

This includes including a combination of fruits, vegetables, protein sources (such as nuts or seeds), and healthy fats (such as avocado or coconut oil).

Overall, the principles of liver detox smoothies revolve around nourishing the body with nutrient-dense, anti-inflammatory ingredients that support liver function and promote detoxification for optimal health.

Benefits of Liver Detox Smoothie

Liver detox smoothies offer a multitude of benefits for overall health and well-being, primarily by supporting liver function and promoting detoxification processes within the body. Here are some key advantages:

Enhanced Liver Function: Liver detox smoothies are designed to provide a concentrated dose of nutrients that support the liver's natural detoxification pathways. Ingredients like leafy greens, fruits, and herbs contain antioxidants and vitamins that help the liver process toxins more efficiently.

Detoxification Support: By including ingredients with detoxifying properties such as chlorophyll-rich greens, citrus fruits, and herbs like cilantro and parsley, liver detox smoothies aid in the removal of harmful toxins and heavy metals from the body, promoting overall detoxification.

Reduced Inflammation: Many ingredients commonly found in liver detox smoothies, such as ginger, turmeric, and omega-3 fatty acids, possess anti-inflammatory properties. Consuming these ingredients regularly can help reduce inflammation in the body, which is beneficial for liver health and overall well-being.

Improved Digestive Health: Liver detox smoothies often contain fiber-rich ingredients like fruits, vegetables, and seeds, which support digestive health and promote regular bowel movements. A healthy digestive system is essential for optimal liver function and overall health.

Boosted Energy Levels: Nutrient-dense ingredients in liver detox smoothies provide a natural energy boost, helping to combat fatigue and support overall vitality.

By nourishing the body with essential vitamins and minerals, these smoothies contribute to increased energy levels and improved stamina throughout the day.

Incorporating liver detox smoothies into your diet can be a delicious and convenient way to support liver health, promote detoxification, and enhance overall well-being.

Tips on Liver Detox Smoothie

Include Liver-Friendly Ingredients: Focus on incorporating ingredients that are known to support liver health, such as leafy greens (like spinach and kale), citrus fruits (like lemon and lime), and herbs (such as parsley and cilantro).

Opt for Organic Produce: When possible, choose organic fruits and vegetables to minimize exposure to pesticides and other harmful chemicals that can burden the liver.

Balance Your Ingredients: Aim for a balanced combination of fruits, vegetables, protein sources (such as nuts or seeds), and healthy fats (like avocado or coconut oil) to ensure your smoothie provides a comprehensive range of nutrients.

Add Detoxifying Herbs and Spices: Incorporate detoxifying herbs and spices like ginger, turmeric, and cinnamon, which can help support the liver's natural detoxification processes and reduce inflammation in the body.

Hydrate Properly: Use a liquid base like water, coconut water, or unsweetened almond milk to blend your smoothie and ensure proper hydration, which is essential for liver health and overall well-being.

Include Fiber-Rich Ingredients: Fiber helps promote regular bowel movements and aids in the elimination of toxins from the body. Add fiber-rich ingredients like chia seeds, flaxseeds, or psyllium husk to your smoothie for added detoxification support.

Avoid Added Sugars and Artificial Ingredients: Steer clear of processed sugars, artificial sweeteners, and other additives that can contribute to liver congestion and inflammation. Instead, sweeten your smoothie naturally with whole fruits like berries or bananas.

By following these tips, you can create delicious and nutrient-packed liver detox smoothies that support liver health, promote detoxification, and contribute to overall well-being.

Guidelines for Liver Detox Smoothie

When preparing liver detox smoothies, it's essential to follow certain guidelines to ensure they are effective and beneficial for your health:

Select Nutrient-Dense Ingredients: Choose a variety of nutrient-dense fruits and vegetables for your smoothie, focusing on those that support liver health such as leafy greens, beets, carrots, and berries.

Include Liver-Supportive Herbs and Spices: Incorporate herbs and spices known for their liver-supportive properties, such as turmeric, ginger, cilantro, and parsley. These ingredients can aid in detoxification and reduce inflammation in the liver.

Choose Organic Produce: Whenever possible, opt for organic fruits and vegetables to minimize exposure to pesticides and other harmful chemicals that can burden the liver.

Limit Added Sugars: Avoid adding refined sugars or artificial sweeteners to your smoothie, as they can contribute to liver congestion and inflammation. Instead, sweeten your smoothie naturally with whole fruits like bananas or dates.

Include Healthy Fats: Add sources of healthy fats such as avocado, coconut oil, or nuts/seeds to your smoothie. Healthy fats are essential for bile production, which aids in the digestion and elimination of toxins from the liver.

Stay Hydrated: Use a liquid base like water, coconut water, or unsweetened almond milk to ensure proper hydration and support the liver's detoxification processes.

Consider Protein: Including a source of protein in your smoothie, such as Greek yogurt, hemp seeds, or protein powder, can help stabilize blood sugar levels and provide amino acids necessary for liver function.

By following these guidelines, you can create liver detox smoothies that are nutritious, delicious, and supportive of overall liver health and detoxification processes.

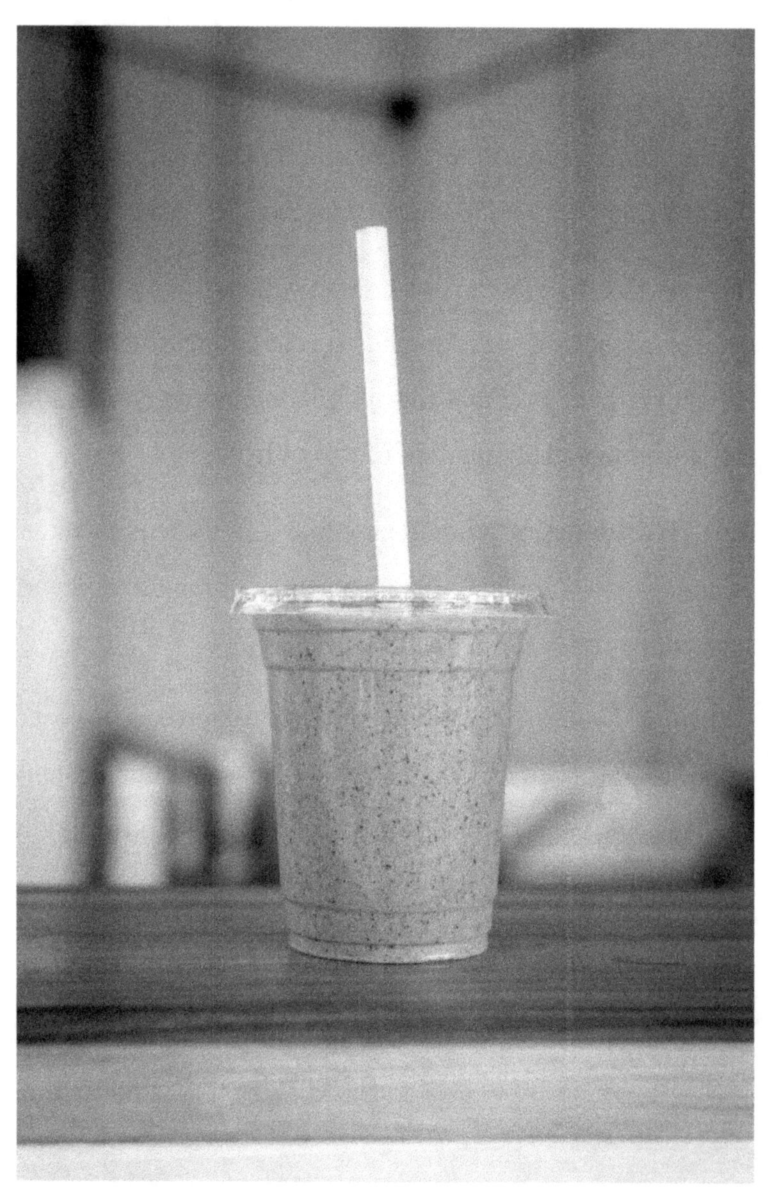

CHAPTER TWO

Liver Detox Smoothie Recipes

1: Green Goddess Detox Smoothie

Ingredients:

- 1 cup spinach
- 1/2 cup kale
- 1/2 cucumber
- 1/2 avocado
- 1/2 lemon (juiced)
- 1 tablespoon fresh ginger (peeled and chopped)
- 1 cup coconut water
- Ice cubes (optional)

Instructions:

- Place all ingredients in a blender.
- Blend until smooth.
- Serve immediately.

Health Benefits:

- This smoothie is packed with chlorophyll-rich greens, healthy fats from avocado, and anti-inflammatory ginger, promoting liver detoxification tion and overall health.

Preparation Time: 5 minutes

2: Berry Beet Detox Smoothie

Ingredients:

- 1/2 cup mixed berries (such as strawberries, blueberries, raspberries)
- 1/2 small beet (peeled and chopped)
- 1/2 cup spinach
- 1 tablespoon chia seeds
- 1 tablespoon fresh lemon juice
- 1 cup almond milk (unsweetened)
- Ice cubes (optional)

Instructions:

- Combine all ingredients in a blender.
- Blend until smooth.
- Enjoy immediately.

Health Benefits:

- This smoothie provides antioxidants from berries, detoxifying properties from beets, fiber from spinach and chia seeds, and hydration from almond milk, supporting liver health and detoxification processes.

Preparation Time: 5 minutes

3: Tropical Turmeric Cleansing Smoothie

Ingredients:

- 1/2 cup pineapple chunks
- 1/2 banana
- 1/2 teaspoon turmeric powder
- 1 tablespoon fresh ginger (peeled and chopped)
- 1 tablespoon coconut oil
- 1 cup coconut water
- Ice cubes (optional)

Instructions:

- Add all ingredients to a blender.
- Blend until smooth.
- Serve immediately.

Health Benefits:

- This smoothie features anti-inflammatory turmeric, digestive-supporting pineapple, immune-boosting ginger, and hydrating coconut water, promoting liver detoxification and overall well-being.

Preparation Time: 5 minutes

4: Citrus Spinach Detox Smoothie

Ingredients:

- ➤ 1/2 cup spinach
- ➤ 1/2 cup kale
- ➤ 1/2 orange (peeled and segmented)
- ➤ 1/2 lemon (juiced)
- ➤ 1 tablespoon fresh mint leaves
- ➤ 1 tablespoon hemp seeds
- ➤ 1 cup water or coconut water
- ➤ Ice cubes (optional)

Instructions:

- ➤ Place all ingredients in a blender.
- ➤ Blend until smooth.
- ➤ Serve immediately.

Health Benefits:

- ➤ This smoothie provides vitamin C from citrus fruits, chlorophyll from leafy greens, detoxifying properties from mint and hemp seeds, and hydration from water or coconut water, supporting liver health and detoxification processes.

Preparation Time: 5 minutes

5: Detoxifying Green Tea Smoothie

Ingredients:

- 1 cup brewed green tea (cooled)
- 1/2 cup spinach
- 1/2 cup cucumber
- 1/2 green apple (cored and chopped)
- 1/4 avocado
- 1 tablespoon fresh lemon juice
- 1 tablespoon honey (optional)
- Ice cubes (optional)

Instructions:

- Combine all ingredients in a blender.
- Blend until smooth.
- Enjoy immediately.

Health Benefits:

- This smoothie features antioxidant-rich green tea, hydrating cucumber, liver-cleansing lemon juice, and fiber from spinach and apple, supporting liver detoxification and overall health.

Preparation Time: 5 minutes

6: Detoxifying Beetroot Smoothie

Ingredients:

- 1/2 small beet (peeled and chopped)
- 1/2 cup frozen berries (such as blueberries or raspberries)
- 1/2 cup spinach
- 1/2-inch fresh ginger (peeled and chopped)
- 1/2 cup coconut water
- 1 tablespoon chia seeds
- Ice cubes (optional)

Instructions:

- Place all ingredients in a blender.
- Blend until smooth.
- Serve immediately.

Health Benefits:

- This smoothie contains detoxifying beets, antioxidant-rich berries, chlorophyll from spinach, digestion-aiding ginger, and hydrating coconut water, supporting liver health and detoxification processes.

Preparation Time: 5 minutes

7: Cleansing Citrus Smoothie

Ingredients:

- 1/2 grapefruit (peeled and segmented)
- 1/2 orange (peeled and segmented)
- 1/2 lemon (juiced)
- 1/2 inch fresh ginger (peeled and chopped)
- 1/2 cup spinach
- 1 tablespoon honey or maple syrup (optional)
- 1 cup water or coconut water
- Ice cubes (optional)

Instructions:

- Combine all ingredients in a blender.
- Blend until smooth.
- Enjoy immediately.

Health Benefits:

- This smoothie features vitamin C-rich citrus fruits, digestion-supporting ginger, chlorophyll from spinach, and hydration from water or coconut water, promoting liver health and detoxification processes.

Preparation Time: 5 minutes

8: Liver-Boosting Blueberry Smoothie

Ingredients:

- 1/2 cup blueberries (fresh or frozen)
- 1/2 cup spinach
- 1/2 cucumber
- 1/2 avocado
- 1 tablespoon fresh lemon juice
- 1 tablespoon flaxseeds
- 1 cup coconut water
- Ice cubes (optional)

Instructions:

- Add all ingredients to a blender.
- Blend until smooth.
- Serve immediately.

Health Benefits:

- This smoothie contains antioxidant-rich blueberries, chlorophyll from spinach, hydrating cucumber and avocado, omega-3 fatty acids from flaxseeds, and hydration from coconut water, supporting liver health and detoxification processes.

Preparation Time: 5 minutes

9: Digestive Detox Smoothie

Ingredients:

- ➤ 1/2 cup pineapple chunks
- ➤ 1/2 cup papaya chunks
- ➤ 1/2 banana
- ➤ 1 tablespoon fresh mint leaves
- ➤ 1/2 inch fresh ginger (peeled and chopped)
- ➤ 1 tablespoon chia seeds
- ➤ 1 cup coconut water
- ➤ Ice cubes (optional)

Instructions:

- ➤ Place all ingredients in a blender.
- ➤ Blend until smooth.
- ➤ Enjoy immediately.

Health Benefits:

> This smoothie features digestion-aiding pineapple and papaya, liver-supporting ginger and mint, fiber-rich chia seeds, and hydration from coconut water, promoting liver health and detoxification processes.

Preparation Time: 5 minutes

10: Superfood Detox Smoothie

Ingredients:

> 1/2 cup mixed berries (such as strawberries, blueberries, raspberries)
> 1/2 cup kale
> 1/2 cup spinach
> 1/2 avocado
> 1 tablespoon spirulina powder
> 1 tablespoon hemp seeds
> 1 cup almond milk (unsweetened)
> Ice cubes (optional)

Instructions:

> Combine all ingredients in a blender.
> Blend until smooth.

- ➤ Serve immediately.

Health Benefits:

- ➤ This smoothie contains antioxidant-rich berries, chlorophyll from kale and spinach, healthy fats from avocado and hemp seeds, and detoxifying spirulina, promoting liver health and overall well-being.

Preparation Time: 5 minutes

11: Carrot Ginger Detox Smoothie

Ingredients:

- ➤ 1/2 cup carrots (peeled and chopped)
- ➤ 1/2 inch fresh ginger (peeled and chopped)
- ➤ 1/2 cup pineapple chunks
- ➤ 1/2 banana
- ➤ 1 tablespoon fresh lemon juice
- ➤ 1 tablespoon honey or maple syrup (optional)
- ➤ 1 cup coconut water or water
- ➤ Ice cubes (optional)

Instructions:

- ➤ Combine all ingredients in a blender.
- ➤ Blend until smooth.

> Serve immediately.

Health Benefits:

> This smoothie features liver-supporting carrots and ginger, digestion-aiding pineapple, hydrating coconut water, and detoxifying lemon juice, promoting liver health and detoxification processes.

Preparation Time: 5 minutes

12: Minty Green Detox Smoothie

Ingredients:

> 1/2 cup cucumber
> 1/2 cup spinach
> 1/2 cup pineapple chunks
> 1/2 banana
> 1 tablespoon fresh mint leaves
> 1 tablespoon chia seeds
> 1 cup coconut water or water
> Ice cubes (optional)

Instructions:

> Add all ingredients to a blender.
> Blend until smooth.

- ➢ Enjoy immediately.

Health Benefits:

- ➢ This smoothie contains hydrating cucumber and pineapple, chlorophyll-rich spinach, digestion-aiding mint, fiber-rich chia seeds, and hydrating coconut water, supporting liver health and detoxification processes.

Preparation Time: 5 minutes

13: Turmeric Mango Detox Smoothie

Ingredients:

- ➢ 1/2 cup mango chunks
- ➢ 1/2 inch fresh turmeric (peeled and chopped) or 1/2 teaspoon turmeric powder
- ➢ 1/2 cup spinach
- ➢ 1/2 cup coconut milk or almond milk (unsweetened)
- ➢ 1 tablespoon honey or maple syrup (optional)
- ➢ Pinch of black pepper (enhances turmeric absorption)
- ➢ Ice cubes (optional)

Instructions:

> Combine all ingredients in a blender.

> Blend until smooth.

> Serve immediately.

Health Benefits:

> This smoothie features anti-inflammatory turmeric, vitamin C-rich mango, chlorophyll from spinach, healthy fats from coconut milk, and digestion-aiding honey, promoting liver health and detoxification processes.

Preparation Time: 5 minutes

14: Beet Detox Smoothie Bowl

Ingredients:

> 1/2 small beet (peeled and chopped)

> 1/2 cup mixed berries (such as strawberries, blueberries, raspberries)

> 1/2 banana

> 1/2 cup spinach

> 1 tablespoon chia seeds

> 1/4 cup Greek yogurt (unsweetened)

- ➢ 1/4 cup almond milk (unsweetened)

- ➢ Ice cubes (optional)

- ➢ Toppings: sliced fruits, nuts/seeds, coconut flakes

Instructions:

- ➢ Place all ingredients (except toppings) in a blender.

- ➢ Blend until smooth.

- ➢ Pour into a bowl and add desired toppings.

- ➢ Enjoy immediately with a spoon.

Health Benefits:

- ➢ This smoothie bowl contains detoxifying beets and berries, fiber-rich spinach and chia seeds, probiotics from Greek yogurt, and hydration from almond milk, promoting liver health and detoxification processes.

Preparation Time: 5 minutes

15: Avocado Detox Green Smoothie

Ingredients:

- ➢ 1/2 avocado

- ➢ 1/2 cup cucumber

- ➢ 1/2 cup spinach

- ➢ 1/2 cup pineapple chunks

> 1 tablespoon fresh lemon juice

> 1 tablespoon fresh parsley leaves

> 1 cup coconut water or water

> Ice cubes (optional)

Instructions:

> Add all ingredients to a blender.

> Blend until smooth.

> Serve immediately.

Health Benefits:

> This smoothie features liver-supporting avocado and cucumber, chlorophyll-rich spinach and parsley, digestion-aiding pineapple, hydrating coconut water, and detoxifying lemon juice, promoting liver health and detoxification processes.

Preparation Time: 5 minutes

16: Kiwi Kale Detox Smoothie

Ingredients:

> 1/2 kiwi (peeled and sliced)

> 1/2 cup kale

> 1/2 cup cucumber

- ➢ 1/2 green apple (cored and chopped)
- ➢ 1 tablespoon fresh lemon juice
- ➢ 1 tablespoon hemp seeds
- ➢ 1 cup coconut water or water
- ➢ Ice cubes (optional)

Instructions:

- ➢ Combine all ingredients in a blender.
- ➢ Blend until smooth.
- ➢ Enjoy immediately.

Health Benefits:

- ➢ This smoothie contains vitamin C-rich kiwi and lemon, chlorophyll from kale, hydration from cucumber and coconut water, omega-3 fatty acids from hemp seeds, and detoxifying properties, supporting liver health and detoxification processes.

Preparation Time: 5 minutes

17: Pineapple Ginger Detox Smoothie

Ingredients:

- ➢ 1/2 cup pineapple chunks
- ➢ 1/2 inch fresh ginger (peeled and chopped)

- ➤ 1/2 cup spinach

- ➤ 1/2 cup cucumber

- ➤ 1/4 avocado

- ➤ 1 tablespoon fresh lime juice

- ➤ 1 cup coconut water or water

- ➤ Ice cubes (optional)

Instructions:

- ➤ Add all ingredients to a blender.

- ➤ Blend until smooth.

- ➤ Serve immediately.

Health Benefits:

- ➤ This smoothie features digestion-aiding pineapple and ginger, chlorophyll from spinach, hydrating cucumber, healthy fats from avocado, detoxifying lime juice, and hydration from coconut water, supporting liver health and detoxification processes.

Preparation Time: 5 minutes

18: Blueberry Kale Detox Smoothie

Ingredients:

- ➤ 1/2 cup blueberries (fresh or frozen)

- ➢ 1/2 cup kale
- ➢ 1/2 banana
- ➢ 1/2 cup cucumber
- ➢ 1 tablespoon fresh lemon juice
- ➢ 1 tablespoon chia seeds
- ➢ 1 cup coconut water or water
- ➢ Ice cubes (optional)

Instructions:

- ➢ Combine all ingredients in a blender.
- ➢ Blend until smooth.
- ➢ Enjoy immediately.

Health Benefits:

- ➢ This smoothie contains antioxidant-rich blueberries, chlorophyll from kale, digestion-aiding cucumber, detoxifying lemon juice, fiber-rich chia seeds, and hydration from coconut water, supporting liver health and detoxification processes.

Preparation Time: 5 minutes

19: Mango Coconut Detox Smoothie

Ingredients:

- ➢ 1/2 cup mango chunks
- ➢ 1/2 banana
- ➢ 1/4 cup coconut flakes
- ➢ 1/4 cup Greek yogurt (unsweetened)
- ➢ 1 tablespoon fresh lime juice
- ➢ 1 tablespoon honey or maple syrup (optional)
- ➢ 1 cup coconut water or water
- ➢ Ice cubes (optional)

Instructions:

- ➢ Add all ingredients to a blender.
- ➢ Blend until smooth.
- ➢ Serve immediately.

Health Benefits:

- ➢ This smoothie features vitamin C-rich mango and lime, hydrating coconut flakes and coconut water, probiotics from Greek yogurt, and digestion-aiding honey, promoting liver health and detoxification processes.

Preparation Time: 5 minutes

20: Apple Spinach Detox Smoothie

Ingredients:

- 1/2 green apple (cored and chopped)
- 1/2 cup spinach
- 1/2 cucumber
- 1/2 inch fresh ginger (peeled and chopped)
- 1 tablespoon fresh lemon juice
- 1 tablespoon hemp seeds
- 1 cup coconut water or water
- Ice cubes (optional)

Instructions:

- Combine all ingredients in a blender.
- Blend until smooth.
- Enjoy immediately.

Health Benefits:

- This smoothie features digestion-aiding apple and ginger, chlorophyll from spinach, hydrating cucumber, detoxifying lemon juice, omega-3 fatty acids from hemp seeds, and hydration from coconut water, supporting liver health and detoxification processes.

Preparation Time: 5 minutes

21: Peach Ginger Detox Smoothie

Ingredients:

- ➢ 1/2 cup sliced peaches (fresh or frozen)
- ➢ 1/2 inch fresh ginger (peeled and chopped)
- ➢ 1/2 cup spinach
- ➢ 1/2 cup cucumber
- ➢ 1/4 avocado
- ➢ 1 tablespoon fresh lemon juice
- ➢ 1 tablespoon honey or maple syrup (optional)
- ➢ 1 cup coconut water or water
- ➢ Ice cubes (optional)

Instructions:

- ➢ Add all ingredients to a blender.
- ➢ Blend until smooth.
- ➢ Serve immediately.

Health Benefits:

> ➤ This smoothie features digestion-aiding peach and ginger, chlorophyll from spinach, hydrating cucumber, healthy fats from avocado, detoxifying lemon juice, and hydration from coconut water, supporting liver health and detoxification processes.

Preparation Time: 5 minutes

22: Pineapple Mango Detox Smoothie

Ingredients:

> ➤ 1/2 cup pineapple chunks
> ➤ 1/2 cup mango chunks
> ➤ 1/2 banana
> ➤ 1/2 cup spinach
> ➤ 1 tablespoon fresh lime juice
> ➤ 1 tablespoon chia seeds
> ➤ 1 cup coconut water or water
> ➤ Ice cubes (optional)

Instructions:

> ➤ Combine all ingredients in a blender.
> ➤ Blend until smooth.

> Enjoy immediately.

Health Benefits:

> This smoothie contains digestion-aiding pineapple and mango, chlorophyll from spinach, detoxifying lime juice, fiber-rich chia seeds, and hydration from coconut water, supporting liver health and detoxification processes.

Preparation Time: 5 minutes

23: Citrus Detox Green Smoothie

Ingredients:

> 1/2 orange (peeled and segmented)
> 1/2 cup pineapple chunks
> 1/2 cup spinach
> 1/2 cucumber
> 1 tablespoon fresh mint leaves
> 1 tablespoon chia seeds
> 1 cup coconut water or water
> Ice cubes (optional)

Instructions:

> Add all ingredients to a blender.

- Blend until smooth.
- Serve immediately.

Health Benefits:

- This smoothie features vitamin C-rich citrus and pineapple, chlorophyll from spinach, digestion-aiding cucumber, detoxifying mint, fiber-rich chia seeds, and hydration from coconut water, supporting liver health and detoxification processes.

Preparation Time: 5 minutes

24: Mango Turmeric Detox Smoothie

Ingredients:

- 1/2 cup mango chunks
- 1/2-inch fresh turmeric (peeled and chopped) or 1/2 teaspoon turmeric powder
- 1/2 cup spinach
- 1/2 cup coconut milk or almond milk (unsweetened)
- 1 tablespoon honey or maple syrup (optional)
- Pinch of black pepper (enhances turmeric absorption)
- Ice cubes (optional)

Instructions:

> ➤ Combine all ingredients in a blender.

> ➤ Blend until smooth.

> ➤ Serve immediately.

Health Benefits:

> ➤ This smoothie features anti-inflammatory turmeric, vitamin C-rich mango, chlorophyll from spinach, healthy fats from coconut milk, and digestion-aiding honey, promoting liver health and detoxification processes.

Preparation Time: 5 minutes

25: Papaya Pineapple Detox Smoothie

Ingredients:

> ➤ 1/2 cup papaya chunks

> ➤ 1/2 cup pineapple chunks

> ➤ 1/2 cup kale

> ➤ 1/2 cucumber

> ➤ 1 tablespoon fresh lime juice

> ➤ 1 tablespoon hemp seeds

> ➤ 1 cup coconut water or water

- ➢ Ice cubes (optional)

Instructions:

- ➢ Add all ingredients to a blender.
- ➢ Blend until smooth.
- ➢ Enjoy immediately.

Health Benefits:

- ➢ This smoothie features digestion-aiding papaya and pineapple, chlorophyll from kale, hydrating cucumber, detoxifying lime juice, omega-3 fatty acids from hemp seeds, and hydration from coconut water, supporting liver health and detoxification processes.

Preparation Time: 5 minutes

26: Berry Spinach Detox Smoothie

Ingredients:

- ➢ 1/2 cup mixed berries (such as strawberries, blueberries, raspberries)
- ➢ 1/2 cup spinach
- ➢ 1/2 cucumber
- ➢ 1/2 banana

- ➤ 1 tablespoon fresh lemon juice
- ➤ 1 tablespoon chia seeds
- ➤ 1 cup coconut water or water
- ➤ Ice cubes (optional)

Instructions:

- ➤ Combine all ingredients in a blender.
- ➤ Blend until smooth.
- ➤ Serve immediately.

Health Benefits:

- ➤ This smoothie contains antioxidant-rich berries, chlorophyll from spinach, digestion-aiding cucumber, detoxifying lemon juice, fiber-rich chia seeds, and hydration from coconut water, supporting liver health and detoxification processes.

Preparation Time: 5 minutes

27: Kiwi Coconut Detox Smoothie

Ingredients:

- ➤ 1/2 kiwi (peeled and sliced)
- ➤ 1/2 cup spinach
- ➤ 1/2 cup coconut flakes

- ➢ 1/2 cucumber
- ➢ 1 tablespoon fresh lime juice
- ➢ 1 tablespoon honey or maple syrup (optional)
- ➢ 1 cup coconut water or water
- ➢ Ice cubes (optional)

Instructions:

- ➢ Add all ingredients to a blender.
- ➢ Blend until smooth.
- ➢ Serve immediately.

Health Benefits:

- ➢ This smoothie features vitamin C-rich kiwi and lime, chlorophyll from spinach, hydrating coconut flakes and cucumber, digestion-aiding honey, and hydration from coconut water, supporting liver health and detoxification processes.

Preparation Time: 5 minutes

28: Blueberry Lemon Detox Smoothie

Ingredients:

- ➢ 1/2 cup blueberries (fresh or frozen)
- ➢ 1/2 cup spinach

- ➢ 1/2 cucumber
- ➢ 1/2 banana
- ➢ 1 tablespoon fresh lemon juice
- ➢ 1 tablespoon hemp seeds
- ➢ 1 cup coconut water or water
- ➢ Ice cubes (optional)

Instructions:

- ➢ Combine all ingredients in a blender.
- ➢ Blend until smooth.
- ➢ Enjoy immediately.

Health Benefits:

- ➢ This smoothie features antioxidant-rich blueberries, chlorophyll from spinach, digestion-aiding cucumber, detoxifying lemon juice, omega-3 fatty acids from hemp seeds, and hydration from coconut water, supporting liver health and detoxification processes.

Preparation Time: 5 minutes

29: Papaya Ginger Detox Smoothie

Ingredients:

- ➢ 1/2 cup papaya chunks
- ➢ 1/2 inch fresh ginger (peeled and chopped)
- ➢ 1/2 cup spinach
- ➢ 1/2 cucumber
- ➢ 1 tablespoon fresh lime juice
- ➢ 1 tablespoon chia seeds
- ➢ 1 cup coconut water or water
- ➢ Ice cubes (optional)

Instructions:

- ➢ Add all ingredients to a blender.
- ➢ Blend until smooth.
- ➢ Serve immediately.

Health Benefits:

- ➢ This smoothie features digestion-aiding papaya and ginger, chlorophyll from spinach, hydrating cucumber, detoxifying lime juice, fiber-rich chia seeds, and hydration from coconut water, supporting liver health and detoxification processes.

Preparation Time: 5 minutes

30: Raspberry Coconut Detox Smoothie

Ingredients:

- 1/2 cup raspberries (fresh or frozen)
- 1/2 cup spinach
- 1/2 cucumber
- 1/4 cup coconut flakes
- 1 tablespoon fresh lemon juice
- 1 tablespoon honey or maple syrup (optional)
- 1 cup coconut water or water
- Ice cubes (optional)

Instructions:

- Combine all ingredients in a blender.
- Blend until smooth.
- Enjoy immediately.

Health Benefits:

- This smoothie features antioxidant-rich raspberries, chlorophyll from spinach, digestion-aiding cucumber, hydrating coconut flakes, detoxifying lemon juice, and digestion-aiding honey, supporting liver health and detoxification processes.

Preparation Time: 5 minutes

31: Pineapple Papaya Detox Smoothie

Ingredients:

- 1/2 cup pineapple chunks
- 1/2 cup papaya chunks
- 1/2 cucumber
- 1/2 banana
- 1 tablespoon fresh lime juice
- 1 tablespoon chia seeds
- 1 cup coconut water or water
- Ice cubes (optional)

Instructions:

- Combine all ingredients in a blender.
- Blend until smooth.
- Serve immediately.

Health Benefits:

- This smoothie features digestion-aiding pineapple and papaya, hydrating cucumber, detoxifying lime juice, fiber-rich chia seeds, and hydration from coconut water, supporting liver health and detoxification processes.

Preparation Time: 5 minutes

32: Mango Mint Detox Smoothie

Ingredients:

- ➢ 1/2 cup mango chunks
- ➢ 1/2 banana
- ➢ 1/4 cup fresh mint leaves
- ➢ 1/2 cucumber
- ➢ 1 tablespoon fresh lime juice
- ➢ 1 tablespoon honey or maple syrup (optional)
- ➢ 1 cup coconut water or water
- ➢ Ice cubes (optional)

Instructions:

- ➢ Add all ingredients to a blender.
- ➢ Blend until smooth.
- ➢ Enjoy immediately.

Health Benefits:

> This smoothie features digestion-aiding mango and cucumber, detoxifying lime juice, refreshing mint, hydration from coconut water, and digestion-aiding honey, supporting liver health and detoxification processes.

Preparation Time: 5 minutes

33: Kiwi Berry Detox Smoothie

Ingredients:

> 1/2 kiwi (peeled and sliced)
> 1/2 cup mixed berries (such as strawberries, blueberries, raspberries)
> 1/2 cucumber
> 1/2 cup spinach
> 1 tablespoon fresh lemon juice
> 1 tablespoon chia seeds
> 1 cup coconut water or water
> Ice cubes (optional)

Instructions:

> Combine all ingredients in a blender.

- ➢ Blend until smooth.
- ➢ Serve immediately.

Health Benefits:

- ➢ This smoothie features vitamin C-rich kiwi and berries, hydrating cucumber, chlorophyll from spinach, detoxifying lemon juice, fiber-rich chia seeds, and hydration from coconut water, supporting liver health and detoxification processes.

Preparation Time: 5 minutes

34: Blueberry Beet Detox Smoothie

Ingredients:

- ➢ 1/2 cup blueberries (fresh or frozen)
- ➢ 1/2 small beet (peeled and chopped)
- ➢ 1/2 cucumber
- ➢ 1/2 cup spinach
- ➢ 1 tablespoon fresh lemon juice
- ➢ 1 tablespoon hemp seeds
- ➢ 1 cup coconut water or water
- ➢ Ice cubes (optional)

Instructions:

> Add all ingredients to a blender.

> Blend until smooth.

> Enjoy immediately.

Health Benefits:

> This smoothie features antioxidant-rich blueberries, detoxifying beets, hydrating cucumber, chlorophyll from spinach, detoxifying lemon juice, omega-3 fatty acids from hemp seeds, and hydration from coconut water, supporting liver health and detoxification processes.

Preparation Time: 5 minutes

35: Pineapple Turmeric Detox Smoothie

Ingredients:

> 1/2 cup pineapple chunks

> 1/2 inch fresh turmeric (peeled and chopped) or 1/2 teaspoon turmeric powder

> 1/2 cucumber

> 1/2 cup spinach

> 1 tablespoon fresh lemon juice

➢ 1 tablespoon honey or maple syrup (optional)

➢ 1 cup coconut water or water

➢ Ice cubes (optional)

Instructions:

➢ Combine all ingredients in a blender.

➢ Blend until smooth.

➢ Serve immediately.

Health Benefits:

➢ This smoothie features digestion-aiding pineapple, anti-inflammatory turmeric, hydrating cucumber, chlorophyll from spinach, detoxifying lemon juice, and digestion-aiding honey, supporting liver health and detoxification processes.

Preparation Time: 5 minutes

36: Raspberry Lemon Detox Smoothie

Ingredients:

➢ 1/2 cup raspberries (fresh or frozen)

➢ 1/2 cucumber

➢ 1/2 cup spinach

➢ 1/2 banana

- ➢ 1 tablespoon fresh lemon juice

- ➢ 1 tablespoon chia seeds

- ➢ 1 cup coconut water or water

- ➢ Ice cubes (optional)

Instructions:

- ➢ Add all ingredients to a blender.

- ➢ Blend until smooth.

- ➢ Enjoy immediately.

Health Benefits:

- ➢ This smoothie features antioxidant-rich raspberries, hydrating cucumber, chlorophyll from spinach, detoxifying lemon juice, fiber-rich chia seeds, and hydration from coconut water, supporting liver health and detoxification processes.

Preparation Time: 5 minutes

37: Mango Coconut Detox Smoothie

Ingredients:

- ➢ 1/2 cup mango chunks

- ➢ 1/2 cucumber

- ➢ 1/2 cup spinach

- 1/4 cup coconut flakes

- 1 tablespoon fresh lime juice

- 1 tablespoon honey or maple syrup (optional)

- 1 cup coconut water or water

- Ice cubes (optional)

Instructions:

- Combine all ingredients in a blender.

- Blend until smooth.

- Serve immediately.

Health Benefits:

- This smoothie features digestion-aiding mango and cucumber, hydrating coconut flakes, chlorophyll from spinach, detoxifying lime juice, digestion-aiding honey, and hydration from coconut water, supporting liver health and detoxification processes.

Preparation Time: 5 minutes

38: Berry Beet Detox Smoothie

Ingredients:

- 1/2 cup mixed berries (such as strawberries, blueberries, raspberries)

- ➢ 1/2 small beet (peeled and chopped)
- ➢ 1/2 cucumber
- ➢ 1/2 cup spinach
- ➢ 1 tablespoon fresh lemon juice
- ➢ 1 tablespoon chia seeds
- ➢ 1 cup coconut water or water
- ➢ Ice cubes (optional)

Instructions:

- ➢ Add all ingredients to a blender.
- ➢ Blend until smooth.
- ➢ Enjoy immediately.

Health Benefits:

- ➢ This smoothie features antioxidant-rich berries, detoxifying beets, hydrating cucumber, chlorophyll from spinach, detoxifying lemon juice, fiber-rich chia seeds, and hydration from coconut water, supporting liver health and detoxification processes.

Preparation Time: 5 minutes

Ingredients:

- 1/2 cup brewed green tea (cooled)
- 1/2 cucumber
- 1/2 cup pineapple chunks
- 1/2 cup spinach
- 1/2-inch fresh ginger (peeled and chopped)
- 1 tablespoon fresh lemon juice
- 1 tablespoon honey or maple syrup (optional)
- Ice cubes (optional)

Instructions:

- Combine all ingredients in a blender.
- Blend until smooth.
- Serve immediately.

Health Benefits:

- This smoothie features antioxidant-rich green tea, hydrating cucumber, digestion-aiding pineapple, chlorophyll from spinach, digestion-supporting ginger, detoxifying lemon juice, and digestion-aiding honey, supporting liver health and detoxification processes.

Preparation Time: 5 minutes

40: Coconut Kale Detox Smoothie

Ingredients:

- ➢ 1/2 cup coconut water or coconut milk
- ➢ 1/2 cup kale
- ➢ 1/2 cucumber
- ➢ 1/2 avocado
- ➢ 1/2 banana
- ➢ 1 tablespoon fresh lime juice
- ➢ 1 tablespoon chia seeds
- ➢ Ice cubes (optional)

Instructions:

- ➢ Add all ingredients to a blender.
- ➢ Blend until smooth.
- ➢ Serve immediately.

Health Benefits:

- ➢ This smoothie features hydrating coconut water or coconut milk, chlorophyll from kale, digestion-aiding cucumber, healthy fats from avocado, digestion-supporting banana, detoxifying lime juice, fiber-rich chia seeds, supporting liver health and detoxification processes.

Preparation Time: 5 minutes

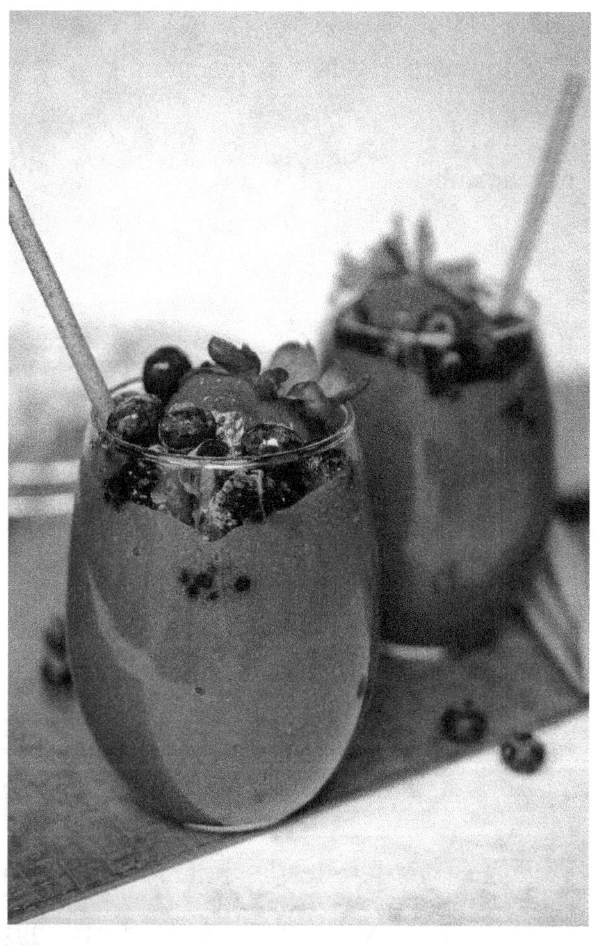

CONCLUSION

Integrating liver detox smoothies into your daily routine can be a delicious and effective way to support your liver health and overall well-being.

These nutrient-packed concoctions offer a plethora of benefits, from detoxifying properties to hydration and essential nutrients.

By incorporating a variety of ingredients such as leafy greens, fruits, herbs, and seeds, you can provide your body with the tools it needs to promote optimal liver function and aid in the detoxification process.

Whether you're looking to kickstart a healthier lifestyle, boost your energy levels, or simply give your liver a well-deserved break, these smoothie recipes offer a convenient and enjoyable solution.

From tangy citrus blends to sweet and refreshing fruit combinations, there's a smoothie recipe to suit every taste preference.

Remember to listen to your body and adjust the ingredients to meet your individual needs and preferences.

Experiment with different flavors and ingredients to keep things exciting and enjoyable.

With regular consumption of these liver detox smoothies, you can embark on a journey towards improved health and vitality.

So, why wait? Start blending up these vibrant concoctions today and give your liver the nourishment it deserves.

Here's to your health and wellness!

www.ingramcontent.com/pod-product-compliance
Lightning Source LLC
Chambersburg PA
CBHW050855260726
48660CB00006B/2642